DIETING COOKBOOK FOR COLON CANCER

The Homemade Nourshing Cancer-Fighting
Recipes for Management and Recovery

TABLE OF CONTENT

INTRODUCTION

Understanding the nuances of our bodies, the impact of our choices, and the potential of holistic approaches to wellness lays the foundation for informed decisions. It is in the realm of understanding, learning, and embracing the intricacies of our bodies that the journey towards improved health truly begins.

Nourishing our bodies is not just about the physical act of consuming food; it is a journey, a continuous exploration of the relationship between what we eat and how we feel. Through these pages, you'll discover the transformative power of nutrient-rich foods and the positive impact they can have on your body.

This book is a beacon, offering insights and practical solutions to navigate the challenges posed by colon cancer. This book is not just a compilation of recipes; it is a thoughtful and purposeful guide crafted to accompany you on a transformative voyage. Every page of this book has been carefully crafted with a singular purpose to guide you on a path of nourishment, resilience, and empowerment. It goes beyond being a mere collection of recipes; it is a holistic approach to wellness that recognizes the interconnectedness of nutrition, immune support, and the fight against cancer cells.

Remember, in the face of health challenges, resilience becomes a guiding force. That why this book also aims to empower you with the knowledge and tools to foster resilience in your journey. As you turn the pages of this book may you find inspiration, knowledge, and a renewed sense of control over your health. This is not just a cookbook; it's a companion on your path to wellness, reminding you that your choices matter and that every meal can be a step towards a healthier and more vibrant life.

CHAPTER ONE

COLON CANCER

Colon cancer, also known as colorectal cancer, is a type of cancer that begins in the large intestine (colon) or rectum. The colon and rectum are part of the digestive system, and their main function is to absorb water and nutrients from food and form waste products (stool).

Colon cancer typically starts as small, noncancerous clumps of cells called polyps. Over time, some of these polyps can develop into colon cancer.

Colon cancer, is a pervasive and potentially life-altering condition which casts a significant shadow on the landscape of health.

This formidable ailment takes root in the large intestine or colon, instigated by the insidious proliferation of abnormal cells that gradually coalesce into tumors along the colon's lining.

The inception of colon cancer frequently emanates from seemingly innocuous benign polyps, which, given time, have the propensity to evolve into cancerous entities, posing a profound threat to an individual's well-being.

The implications of colon cancer extend beyond the confines of a singular organ, permeating various facets of health. Digestion, a cornerstone of physiological equilibrium, becomes a battleground as the malignant presence disrupts the normal functioning of the colon.

The very process of nutrient absorption, essential for sustaining bodily functions, is impeded, further exacerbating the multifaceted impact of this condition.

As the body contends with the encroachment of cancerous cells, overall well-being becomes a precarious balance, with each aspect of health intertwined in the intricate dance with this formidable adversary.

Several factors can increase the risk of developing colon cancer. These includes; Age, Family history, Personal history of colorectal cancer or polyps, Inflammatory bowel diseases, Inherited syndromes and Lifestyle factors

While some risk factors are beyond control, there are several strategies to reduce the risk of colon cancer which includes;

- Regular screenings, such as colonoscopies, can detect and remove precancerous polyps.
- Adopting a diet rich in fruits, vegetables, and whole grains while minimizing red and processed meats. Regular exercise and maintaining a healthy weight are also crucial.
- Limiting alcohol intake can contribute to reducing the risk.
- Quitting smoking is beneficial for overall health and can lower the risk of colon cancer.

NUTRITION AND COLON CANCER

Nutrition stands as a cornerstone in the intricate web of factors influencing health, especially when one is navigating the challenging terrain of cancer treatment. The symbiotic relationship between nutrition and the immune system becomes particularly crucial during this journey, as the body's capacity to combat cancer cells and recuperate from rigorous treatments is intricately linked to the array of nutrients it receives.

A well-balanced and nutrient-rich diet emerges as a linchpin in this narrative, offering a multifaceted approach to supporting the immune system. The holistic benefits extend beyond the immediate concerns of cancer treatment, encompassing the broader spectrum of well-being.

Such a diet not only aids in managing the often arduous side effects of cancer treatments but also serves as a catalyst in enhancing energy levels, fostering resilience, and promoting overall health.

In the realm of immune support, certain nutrients emerge as stalwarts, championing the body's defense mechanisms. Antioxidants, renowned for their ability to neutralize harmful free radicals, form a frontline defense against oxidative stress, a common occurrence during cancer treatment.

Meanwhile, vitamins and minerals act as vital co-factors in numerous physiological processes, orchestrating the intricate dance of cellular functions that underpin a robust immune response.

Scientific evidence underscores the pivotal role of nutrition in fortifying the body's immune arsenal.

Beyond the immediate benefits of alleviating treatment-related side effects, a nutrient-rich diet lays the groundwork for the prevention of illness and, in some cases, the potential hindrance of cancer cell proliferation.

It's a proactive stance towards health, acknowledging that the body's innate resilience is fueled by the quality and diversity of nutrients it receives.

In essence, the journey through cancer treatment is not solely a medical endeavor but a holistic expedition where nutrition emerges as a potent ally.

The incorporation of a well-balanced, nutrient-rich diet becomes a tangible expression of self-care, resilience, and a profound investment in the body's capacity to withstand and overcome the challenges inherent in the fight against cancer.

Proper nutrition plays a significant role in both managing and preventing colon cancer these include;

- Fiber-rich diet: High-fiber foods, such as fruits, vegetables, and whole grains, help maintain bowel regularity and may lower the risk of colon cancer.
- Calcium and Vitamin D: Adequate intake of calcium and vitamin D, through diet or supplements, may have protective effects against colon cancer.
- Antioxidants: Foods rich in antioxidants, such as fruits and vegetables, help neutralize free radicals that can contribute to cancer development.

- Limiting red and processed meats: Diets high in red and processed meats have been linked to an increased risk of colon cancer.

- Hydration: Staying well-hydrated supports overall digestive health.

HOW TO BOOST YOUR IMMUNITY

An immune system is indispensable during cancer treatment, serving as the body's frontline defense against the growth of cancer cells. The immune system's multifaceted role becomes evident in its ability to identify and eliminate cancer cells, thereby thwarting the progression and dissemination of the disease.

This process is fundamental in preventing the unchecked proliferation of abnormal cells that characterize cancer.

Moreover, a well-functioning immune system goes beyond its role as a vigilant guardian; it actively contributes to the efficacy of cancer treatments such as chemotherapy and immunotherapy. By bolstering the body's immune response, these treatments can be more potent in reducing tumor size and mitigating the risk of cancer recurrence.

Cancer treatments often induce immunosuppression, rendering individuals more susceptible to infections. Strengthening the immune system through proper nutrition emerges as a pivotal strategy to mitigate this risk.

A diet rich in immune-supportive nutrients becomes a cornerstone in fortifying the body's defenses against opportunistic infections.

By providing the necessary building blocks for immune cells and supporting their optimal function, a well-balanced diet becomes a crucial ally in maintaining the overall well-being of individuals navigating the challenging terrain of cancer treatment.

In essence, the significance of a healthy immune system during cancer treatment extends far beyond conventional notions of defense; it actively participates in the therapeutic journey, influencing treatment outcomes and fortifying the body against the collateral vulnerabilities induced by cancer therapies.

FOODS TYPES FOR COLON CANCER

High-fiber foods play a pivotal role in promoting digestive health and reducing the risk of colorectal cancer.

Emphasizing the importance of fiber in the diet, particularly through the inclusion of whole grains like oats, quinoa, and brown rice, helps regulate bowel movements.

Fiber acts as a natural bulking agent, facilitating the smooth passage of stool through the digestive tract. This not only alleviates constipation but also contributes to a healthier colon environment. In addition to whole grains, incorporating legumes, fruits, and vegetables into one's daily meals enhances the fiber content.

These foods provide a spectrum of soluble and insoluble fibers, each with its unique benefits. Soluble fiber, found in fruits like apples and citrus, helps lower cholesterol levels, while insoluble fiber, abundant in vegetables such as broccoli and carrots, aids in maintaining bowel regularity.

A colorful array of fruits and vegetables further augments the nutritional profile of a cancer-fighting diet. Berries, with their vibrant hues, are rich in antioxidants like anthocyanins, known for their potential in preventing cell damage and inflammation. Leafy greens, carrots, and tomatoes contribute an array of vitamins, minerals, and phytonutrients, collectively supporting overall well-being and bolstering the body's defense mechanisms against diseases, including colorectal cancer.

Introducing healthy fats into the diet, such as those found in avocados, nuts, and olive oil, is crucial for sustaining various bodily functions. These sources provide essential fatty acids, which not only serve as a concentrated energy source but also aid in the absorption of fat-soluble vitamins like A, D, E, and K. Striking a balance between incorporating these healthy fats and maintaining a diet rich in fiber creates a harmonious approach to supporting digestive and overall health.

In tandem with fiber and healthy fats, lean proteins form an integral component of a well-rounded, cancer-fighting diet. Sources such as fish, poultry, tofu, and legumes supply the body with essential amino acids necessary for cell repair and maintenance.

Choosing lean protein options aligns with the goal of promoting overall health while minimizing saturated fat intake, contributing to a holistic approach in the fight against colorectal cancer.

HOW TO PLAN MEALS FOR OPTIMAL NUTRITION

Have a Mix of Macronutrients;

- Incorporate complex carbohydrates such as whole grains, legumes, and vegetables. These provide a sustained release of energy.

- Include lean protein sources like poultry, fish, tofu, or legumes to support muscle health and repair.

- Choose healthy fats from sources like avocados, nuts, seeds, and olive oil for heart health and satiety.

- Includes variety of Colorful Fruits and Vegetables;

- Different colors indicate different phytonutrients, so aim for a rainbow on your plate. Include leafy greens, berries, citrus fruits, and cruciferous vegetables to maximize nutritional diversity.

Choose Whole Grains;

- Opt for whole grains like brown rice, quinoa, and oats instead of refined grains. Whole grains provide more fiber, vitamins, and minerals. Fiber aids in digestion, helps maintain a healthy weight, and supports overall gut health.

Plan for Regular, Smaller Meals;

- Eating smaller, more frequent meals helps maintain steady blood sugar levels throughout the day. This approach can prevent energy crashes and overeating during main meals. Include healthy snacks by choosing snacks that combine protein and fiber for sustained energy.

- Examples include Greek yogurt with fruit, veggies with hummus, or a handful of nuts.

Incorporate Water and Herbal Teas;

- Water is essential for overall health, aiding in digestion, nutrient absorption, and temperature regulation.
- Herbal teas provide hydration without added calories and can have additional health benefits.

Try Limit Sugary Drinks;

- Sugary beverages can contribute to excess calorie intake and may lead to weight gain. Opt for water, herbal teas, or infused water with slices of fruits for a refreshing, low-calorie option.
- Moderate Caffeine Intake: While moderate caffeine consumption can be

part of a healthy diet, excessive intake may lead to dehydration. Be mindful of your overall caffeine intake and balance it with water consumption.

By paying attention to these aspects, you can create meals that not only taste good but also provide a well-rounded mix of nutrients to support your overall health and well-being.

Tips for Busy Schedules

- Create a weekly meal calendar, outlining each day's breakfast, lunch, dinner, and snacks. This provides a visual guide for the week ahead.

- Establishing theme nights not only adds variety but simplifies the decision-making process. For example, designate a specific night for pasta dishes or stir-fries. This helps streamline your grocery shopping and ensures you have the necessary ingredients on hand.

- Dedicate a specific time to wash, chop, and portion vegetables and fruits for the week. Store them in airtight containers or resealable bags for easy access during daily meal preparation.

- Cook proteins such as chicken, tofu, or lean beef in bulk during your prep session. Portion them into meal-sized containers and refrigerate or freeze. This reduces daily cooking time and provides readily available protein sources.

- Opt for one-pot or sheet pan recipes that allow you to combine multiple ingredients in a single cooking vessel. This minimizes the number of dishes to clean and simplifies the overall cooking process.

- Explore recipes like casseroles, stir-fries, or sheet pan dinners. These not only save time but also allow for creativity in combining flavors and textures within one dish.

- Take advantage of pre-cut vegetables and fruits available at the grocery store. These can significantly reduce preparation time without compromising on freshness.

- Incorporate canned beans and frozen fruits into your meals. They are convenient, have a longer shelf life, and maintain nutritional value. Canned beans can be rinsed and added to salads, while frozen fruits are perfect for smoothies.

- When time is limited, choose wisely from pre-packaged options, such as whole-grain wraps or pre-cooked quinoa. Ensure they align with your nutritional goals and provide a quick and healthy base for your meals.

By incorporating these detailed strategies into your weekly routine, you'll not only save time but also make meal preparation more enjoyable and manageable. Tailor these suggestions to your preferences and dietary requirements for a personalized and efficient approach to healthy eating.

LIFESTYLE TIPS FOR COLON HEALTH

The journey towards colon health extends beyond the confines of the kitchen. While nutrition plays a pivotal role in fortifying the body against the challenges of colon cancer, adopting a holistic approach to your lifestyle is equally crucial.

Incorporating Physical Activity

Regular exercise is not merely a regimen for physical fitness; it emerges as a powerful ally in the battle against colon cancer. Numerous studies have established a compelling link between an active lifestyle and a reduced risk of colon cancer.

A balanced exercise routine should encompass a mix of aerobic activities, such as brisk walking, jogging, or cycling, coupled with strength training exercises.

The synergy of these components contributes not only to overall fitness but also significantly mitigates the risk of colon-related issues. Health guidelines recommend aiming for at least 150 minutes of moderate-intensity exercise per week, and the beauty lies in its flexibility.

Whether in shorter sessions throughout the week or more extended workouts, the key is consistency.

Beyond the apparent physical benefits, regular exercise exerts a profound impact on digestive health. Improved bowel regularity and reduced inflammation are among the notable advantages, promoting an environment in which the colon can function optimally. This serves as a crucial line of defense against potential risks, fortifying the body's resilience.

However, the journey toward a healthier lifestyle need not be arduous. Encouraging readers to find activities they genuinely enjoy is paramount. When exercise becomes an enjoyable pursuit rather than a chore, individuals are more likely to adhere to a consistent routine.

Whether it's dancing, hiking, or engaging in a team sport, the options are diverse, ensuring that there's an activity suited to every preference.

In the pursuit of colon health, let the rhythm of your footsteps or the resistance of weights become a testament to your commitment.

Stress Management Techniques

Chronic stress, an unwelcome companion in our fast-paced lives, can exert profound effects on overall health, with the digestive system bearing a significant brunt. The intricate connection between stress and the digestive system underscores the importance of adopting effective stress management techniques.

- Mindfulness and Meditation

One powerful antidote to the chaos of daily life is the practice of mindfulness and meditation. Encouraging readers to embrace deep breathing exercises, meditation sessions, or the calming embrace of yoga, we aim to guide them toward a state of relaxation.

These practices not only provide a respite from the pressures of the outside world but also trigger physiological responses that counteract the negative impact of stress on the digestive system.

By incorporating mindfulness into their routine, readers can cultivate a sense of calm amidst the storm, promoting not only mental well-being but also digestive health.

- Adequate Sleep for Stress Reduction

The significance of adequate, quality sleep cannot be overstated when it comes to stress reduction and overall well-being.

Lack of sleep not only exacerbates stress levels but also compromises the body's ability to repair and regenerate. Within this discussion, we emphasize the importance of establishing healthy sleep patterns and offer practical tips for improving sleep hygiene.

By prioritizing rest, readers can fortify their resilience against the challenges of daily life, enhancing both mental and digestive health.

- Time Management Strategies

Effective time management is a potent tool in the arsenal against stress. In this segment, we delve into strategies for organizing daily tasks and priorities, providing readers with a roadmap to navigate the demands of their lives.

By fostering a sense of control over their time, individuals can minimize stressors and create a conducive environment for both mental and digestive well-being.

As you explore these stress management techniques, remember that adopting a holistic approach to health involves not only nourishing the body but also nurturing the mind.

By incorporating these practices into their daily lives, readers can take proactive steps towards mitigating the impact of stress on their digestive system, fostering a resilient and balanced life.

CHAPTER TWO

DIETING FOR COLON CANCER

Cancer treatments often bring a slew of side effects that can disrupt daily life. Proper nutrition becomes a powerful ally in managing these challenges.

Specific foods, such as ginger, have been recognized for their ability to alleviate nausea, providing a natural and accessible remedy.

Nutrient-dense foods are instrumental in combating fatigue, a common side effect of many cancer therapies. By tailoring the diet to address these specific concerns, individuals can enhance their quality of life and better endure the rigors of treatment

A well-balanced diet is a cornerstone in the holistic approach to health, particularly when navigating the challenging terrain of cancer treatment. Beyond its direct impact on the immune system, a balanced diet plays a multifaceted role in promoting overall well-being during this critical time. One crucial aspect is the maintenance of a healthy body weight.

A balanced diet ensures that individuals receive the necessary nutrients in the right proportions, aiding in the preservation of a healthy weight.

This is vital for managing energy levels, which can be significantly compromised during cancer treatment. The body's resilience is enhanced when it is adequately fueled and supported, contributing to a more effective response to treatment.

Moreover, the impact of diet extends beyond the physical realm to mental and emotional well-being.

Certain nutrients, including omega-3 fatty acids, have been associated with improved mood and cognitive function. By nourishing the body with foods rich in these essential elements, individuals can foster a positive mindset, resilience, and mental clarity throughout your cancer journey.

Cashew Butter Banana Toast

TOTAL TIME: 10 MINUTES

Ingredients

- ➢ 4 slices of bread
- ➢ 2.5 bananas
- ➢ 2 tbsp cashew butter
- ➢ drizzle of honey
- ➢ sprinkle of cinnamon

Directions

- ➢ Place slices of bread in air fryer at 320-350 for 2 minutes.
- ➢ Line your air fryer with parchment paper and preheat to 375 degrees. Add the banana slices to the air fryer basket, making sure that they do not touch each other. Cook for 5 minutes, or until browned/caramelized.
- ➢ While the bananas are cooking, spread cashew butter over the toast.
- ➢ Top with bananas and add a drizzle of honey + sprinkle of cinnamon.
- ➢ Serve warm!

Balsamic Strawberry Avocado Toast

TOTAL TIME: 5 MINUTES

Ingredients

- ➢ 2 slices whole grain, seeded bread
- ➢ 1 large avocado
- ➢ 6 large strawberries, thinly sliced
- ➢ 1/4 cup feta cheese
- ➢ 1 tbsp balsamic glaze
- ➢ 1/2 tbsp bagel seasoning

Directions

- ➢ Toast the bread to your preferred level of crunch in the toaster or on the stovetop.
- ➢ Meanwhile, slice the avocado and remove the pit. Score with a small knife, then scoop into a small bowl. Mash lightly with the back of a spoon,

then spread onto each slice of the toasted bread.

➢ Top with the sliced strawberries and feta cheese crumbles. Top with a drizzle of the balsamic glaze and bagel seasoning. Serve immediately.

Protein Bars

TOTAL TIME: 2 MINUTES

Ingredients

➢ 1/2 cup coconut flour

➢ 3/4 cup protein powder

➢ 2 cups peanut butter Can sub for any nut or seed butter

➢ 1/2 cup maple syrup

➢ 2 cups chocolate chips Optional

Directions

- ➢ Line a deep pan with parchment paper and set aside. For thicker bars, use an 8 x 8-inch pan. For thinner bars, use any size bigger.

- ➢ In a large mixing bowl, add your dry ingredients and mix well.

- ➢ In a small mixing bowl, melt your peanut butter with sticky sweetener until combined. Add to dry ingredients and mix until fully combined.

- ➢ Transfer protein bar batter into the lined baking dish and press firmly in place. Refrigerate or freeze until firm. Once firm, cut into bars and cover in optional chocolate and enjoy!

Overnight Steel Cut Oats

Ingredients

- 1 ½ cups steel cut oats
- 3 cups water
- 3 cups almond milk
- ½ teaspoon Kosher salt
- 1 banana sliced
- 2 tablespoons creamy peanut butter
- 1 tablespoon peanuts chopped
- Dash of cinnamon
- Strawberry Nutella
- 4-5 strawberries sliced
- 2 tablespoons nutella
- 1 tablespoon hazelnuts chopped
- 1 tablespoon maple syrup
- Caramel Apple
- 1/2 green apple sliced
- 2 tablespoons caramel sauce
- 1 tablespoon pecans chopped

- ➢ Dash of cinnamon

- ➢ Chocolate Almond Butter

- ➢ 2 ounces bittersweet chocolate bar chopped

- ➢ 2 tablespoons almond butter

- ➢ 2 dates chopped

- ➢ 1 tablespoon honey

Directions

- ➢ In a large pot over medium-high heat, bring the water, milk and salt to a boil.

- ➢ Stir in the oats and continue mixing with the liquid for 2-3 minutes to warm up the oats.

- ➢ Turn off the heat, Let it come to room temperature and then store in the fridge overnight.

- ➢ In the morning, heat for a couple minutes while stirring the mixture, and serve with your favorite topping combinations.

Healthy Pumpkin Overnight Oats

TOTAL TIME: 10 MINUTES

Ingredients

- 1/3 cup plain Greek yogurt
- 1/2 cup (heaping) rolled oats
- 2/3 cup unsweetened milk of choice
- 1 tablespoon chia seeds or ground flax meal
- 1/2 teaspoon vanilla extract
- Pinch of salt
- 0–2 tablespoons honey or maple syrup
- 1/2 cup plain pumpkin puree
- 1/2 teaspoon ground cinnamon
- 1/8 teaspoon ground cloves
- 1/4 teaspoon ground nutmeg

Directions

- ➢ Whisk together all ingredients in a medium-sized mixing bowl. Spoon into a jar with a tight-fitting lid.
- ➢ Close and refrigerate for at least 4 hours, but preferably overnight before eating.

Chickpea Caesar Salad

TOTAL TIME: 30 MINUTES

Ingredients

- ➢ 1 batch Tandoori Spiced Chickpeas
- ➢ 2 large bundles lacinato or curly kale, chopped or torn (2 large bundles equals ~16 ounces)
- ➢ 1 Tbsp olive oil
- ➢ 1 Tbsp lemon juice

- 1/4 cup vegan parmesan cheese (optional)
- 2 Tbsp hemp seeds (optional)
- DRESSING
- 1 cup raw cashews (option to soak overnight in cool water, or in hot water for 1 hour)
- 1 tsp dijon mustard
- 1/2 tsp each sea salt and black pepper, plus more to taste
- 8-12 medium cloves fresh garlic, chopped
- 4 tsp capers in brine
- 2 tsp brine juice from capers
- 6 Tbsp lemon juice (2 large lemons yield ~6 Tbsp or 90 ml)
- 3-4 Tbsp olive oil
- 1/2 cup hot water (plus more to thin)
- 1 tsp chickpea (or soy) miso paste

➢ 1 tsp pure maple syrup (or sub Stevia to taste)

Directions

➢ If serving with crispy chickpeas, prepare at this time (see link above).

➢ To prepare dressing, add raw cashews, dijon mustard, salt, pepper, garlic, capers, brine juice (from capers), lemon juice, olive oil, hot water, miso paste, and maple syrup to a small or high-speed blender. Blend until creamy and smooth, scraping down sides as needed. Add enough water to thin until pourable.

➢ Taste and adjust seasonings as needed, adding more lemon or mustard for zing, salt or capers for saltiness, olive oil for creaminess, maple syrup to sweeten, or miso for more depth of flavor. Set aside.

➢ Add kale to a large mixing bowl. Drizzle with 1 Tbsp (15 ml) each olive oil and lemon juice as recipe is written. Massage by hand to remove some of the bitterness and soften the texture.

➢ Add desired amount of dressing, plus vegan parmesan cheese and hemp seeds (both optional). Toss to coat and top with crispy chickpeas. Serve immediately. There may be leftover dressing, which will keep covered in the refrigerator for up to 7-10 days. Not freezer friendly.

Spicy watermelon salad

TOTAL TIME: 25 MINUTES

Ingredients

- 1 cup pumpkin seeds or pepita's
- 1 teaspoon olive oil
- ¾ teaspoon salt
- ½ teaspoon smoked paprika
- ¼ teaspoon cayenne pepper
- Juice from 1 medium lime
- 1/4 of a watermelon cleaned and cubed. Seedless is best here.
- 1/4 cucumber in quarters
- ¼ cup extra-virgin olive oil
- 1 teaspoon chili powder
- ½ teaspoon salt
- ¼ teaspoon cayenne pepper
- 2 medium limes finely grated zest and juice
- 2 tablespoons fresh mint leaves

Directions

➢ Preheat the oven to 180°C (325°F) Mix the pepita's in a bowl with the olive oil, salt, smoked paprika, cayenne and lime juice, Mix it well.

➢ Take a baking tray and line with baking paper. Spread the pepitas out in a single layer and toast for 12 to 15 minutes in the oven.

➢ Let them cool slightly while you make the rest of the salad. You need only a bit for this recipe so keep the rest to nibble on or spread over other dishes. I used them that same night on a poke bowl with chicken.

➢ Combine the watermelon cubes, cucumber, olive oil, chili, salt, lime zest and juice in a bit bowl and mix it all up. Taste and add salt and pepper if needed.

- ➢ Garnish with fresh mint leaves and toasted pepitas. Serve immediately!

Avocado Caprese Salad

TOTAL TIME: 5 MINUTES

INGREDIENTS

- ➢ 8 ounces mozzarella balls (2 medium balls)
- ➢ 3 medium tomatoes
- ➢ 1 avocado
- ➢ 2 tablespoons extra-virgin olive oil
- ➢ 2 tablespoons balsamic reduction
- ➢ kosher salt and freshly ground black pepper to taste
- ➢ handful of fresh basil leaves

Directions

- ➢ Slice the tomatoes, mozzarella, and avocado.

> Alternate slices of the tomatoes, mozzarella, and avocado on a plate. Drizzle with olive oil and balsamic reduction. Sprinkle with salt, pepper, and top with basil leaves.

Broccoli Pasta Salad

TOTAL TIME: 23 MINUTES

Ingredients

> 4 cups broccoli cut into small pieces
>
> 8 ounces rotini pasta or short pasta
>
> ⅓ cup red onion diced
>
> ½ cup dried cranberries
>
> ¼ cup sunflower seeds
>
> 8 slices bacon cooked and crumbled
>
> ½ cup feta cheese optional
>
> 2 teaspoons sugar
>
> 3 tablespoons white wine vinegar
>
> ¾ cup mayonnaise

> ¼ cup sour cream

> salt & pepper

Directions

> Whisk dressing ingredients in a small bowl. Set aside.

> Cook pasta according to package directions. Drain and run under cold water.

> Add remaining ingredients to a larger bowl.

> Pour the prepared dressing over and mix well.

> Refrigerate for one hour before serving.

Avocado Chickpea Salad

TOTAL TIME: 20 MINUTES

INGREDIENTS

- 3 large avocados
- 1 can chickpeas, 15 oz
- 1/2 cup crumbled feta cheese
- 1/4 red onion, thinly sliced
- 2 -3 tbsp fresh parsley or cilantro, chopped
- 1 lemon, juiced
- 1 tsp sumac
- Olive oil
- Salt & pepper
- 1 clove crushed garlic (optional)

DIRECTIONS

- Slice the avocados and add them to a salad bowl.

- ➢ Add in the rinsed chickpeas, sliced onion, feta cheese and chopped cilantro.
- ➢ Generously drizzle with olive oil and pour the lemon juice over the top. Season with the sumac and salt & pepper to taste, and the crushed garlic if using
- ➢ Toss everything together and adjust seasoning if needed. Serve alongside your favorite main course

Simple Kale Salad

TOTAL TIME: 15 MINUTES

Ingredients

For the dressing:

- ➢ 1/4 cup olive oil
- ➢ 2 tablespoons fresh lemon juice
- ➢ 2 tablespoons balsamic vinegar

- ➢ 1/2 teaspoon Dijon mustard
- ➢ 1 to 2 teaspoons honey
- ➢ Kosher salt and freshly ground black pepper, to taste

For the salad:

- ➢ 2 bunches kale, washed (I prefer Lacinato kale)
- ➢ Drizzle of olive oil
- ➢ Pinch of kosher salt
- ➢ 1/2 cup finely shredded Parmesan cheese
- ➢ 1/3 cup toasted sliced almonds, can use pine nuts or pepitas
- ➢ 1/3 cup dried cranberries, can use golden raisins or dried currants

Directions

- ➢ To make the dressing, in a small bowl or jar, whisk together the olive oil, lemon juice, balsamic vinegar, Dijon mustard, honey, salt, and pepper. Set aside.

➢ First, remove the kale stems. Squeeze the top of the kale stem and slowly move your hand down the kale stem. The leafy part of the kale will come right off as you go down. Use a sharp knife to finely chop the kale.

➢ Place the kale in a large bowl. Drizzle the kale with just a little bit of olive oil, you don't need a ton because you are adding a dressing. Sprinkle with a little kosher salt and massage with your clean fingers until the kale softens a bit.

➢ Drizzle the dressing over the kale and toss well. Add the Parmesan cheese, nuts, and dried fruit. Toss again and serve.

Pomegranate and Pear Salad

TOTAL TIME: 15 MINUTES

Ingredients

- 8 cups baby spinach leaves , or mixed greens or arugula
- 2 large ripe pears , cored and sliced
- 1/2 cup pomegranate seeds
- 2 ounces crumbled goat, feta, or gorgonzola cheese
- 1/2 cup slivered almonds, walnuts or pistachios
- For the dressing
- 1/4 cup apple cider vinegar (or champagne vinegar)
- 3 Tablespoons olive oil
- 1 teaspoon dijon mustard
- 1 1/2 Tablespoons honey
- Salt and freshly ground black pepper , to taste

Directions

- ➢ Place all salad ingredients in a large bowl.

- ➢ Make the dressing by whisking all ingredients together.

- ➢ Drizzle dressing over salad and toss to combine. Serve immediately.

Mushroom Barley Soup

TOTAL TIME: 1 HOUR 20 MINUTES

Ingredients

- ➢ 1 cup barley
- ➢ 1 tablespoon olive oil
- ➢ 1 large yellow onion chopped
- ➢ 2 cloves garlic minced
- ➢ 2 carrots peeled and diced
- ➢ 2 celery stalks diced
- ➢ 1 16 oz package of white button mushrooms, sliced

- 3 15 ounce cans low sodium vegetable broth
- 1 cup water
- 2 bay leaves
- 2 tablespoons fresh thyme minced
- Salt and pepper to taste

Directions

- In a medium pan, bring 4 cups of water and the 1 cup of barley to a boil. Cover, reduce heat to medium-low, and simmer for 30-40 minutes, or until the barley is soft. You can make this the night before.
- Heat the olive oil in a large pot over medium heat. Add the onion and garlic. Cook until soft. Add the carrots and celery and cook until tender, about 5 minutes. Add the sliced mushrooms and cook until they are

soft. Add the vegetable broth, water, bay leaves, and fresh thyme. Simmer for about 10 minutes. Stir in the cooked barley and cook for 15 minutes or so.

➢ Remove the bay leaves. Before serving, add salt and pepper to taste. Serve hot.

Pumpkin Curry Soup

TOTAL TIME: 25 MINUTES

Ingredients

➢ 2 teaspoons coconut oil or extra-virgin olive oil

➢ 1 1/2 cups chopped sweet yellow onion about 1 medium

➢ 3 cloves garlic minced (about 1 tablespoon)

➢ 1 tablespoon minced fresh ginger

➢ 3 tablespoons Thai red curry paste

- ➢ 2-3 cups low-sodium vegetable broth or low-sodium chicken broth if the soup being vegetarian is not a concern, divided
- ➢ 2 tablespoons almond butter or peanut butter, I used natural drippy peanut butter
- ➢ 2 cans pure pumpkin puree (15 ounce cans) not pumpkin pie filling
- ➢ 1/2 tablespoon coconut sugar or light brown sugar. Do not omit, as it balances the flavor of the soup
- ➢ 1 teaspoon ground cumin
- ➢ 1/2 teaspoon kosher salt
- ➢ 1/4 teaspoon ground black pepper
- ➢ 1/8 to 1/4 teaspoon cayenne pepper plus additional to taste
- ➢ 1 can light coconut milk (14 ounces)
- ➢ For topping: chopped roasted peanuts or pepitas chopped fresh cilantro,

coconut cream or plain nonfat Greek yogurt

Directions

> In a large pot or Dutch oven, melt the coconut oil over medium heat. Add the onion and sauté for 5 minutes, until translucent. Add the garlic and ginger and cook 1 additional minute, until fragrant. Stir in the Thai curry paste.

> In a small bowl or large measuring cup, whisk together 1/3 cup of the vegetable broth and the almond butter or peanut butter until smooth. Add the mixture to the pot. Add the pumpkin, coconut sugar, cumin, salt, pepper, cayenne, and 1 2/3 cups of the remaining vegetable broth. Stir until well combined.

➢ With an immersion blender, puree the
soup until completely smooth, adding
a little of the coconut milk if it is too
thick to blend smoothly. Alternatively,
you can ladle the soup carefully into a
blender or food processor and puree it
in small batches. Stir in the remaining
coconut milk. If the soup is too thick
for your liking, add additional
vegetable broth until you reach your
desired consistency.

➢ Taste and add additional salt, black
pepper, and/or cayenne pepper as
desired.

Cucumber Soup

Ingredients

- 2 large cucumbers (about 1 1/2 pounds total)
- 2 tablespoons chopped onion (white, red, or green)
- 1/2 cup buttermilk
- 1/4 cup sour cream
- 1 tablespoon rice vinegar
- 1 tablespoon extra virgin olive oil
- 2 tablespoons fresh dill, chopped
- 1/2 teaspoon kosher salt
- Pinch black pepper

Directions

- Prep the cucumbers, onion, and dill:
- Peel, seed, and roughly chop the cucumbers. Chop the onion and dill.

- Put all of the ingredients into a blender and pulse until completely smooth.
- Adjust seasonings to taste. Add more salt and pepper if needed.
- At this point you can make ahead and chill.
- Chill in a container in the refrigerator until cold.
- Pour into bowls and garnish with a drizzle of olive oil and a feather of dill.

Jerk Spiced Minute Steaks with Pineapple Salsa

TOTAL TIME: 55 MINUTES

Ingredients

- 75g brown basmati rice
- 2 top rump minute steaks
- 2 tsp Jamaican jerk seasoning

- ➤ ½ pineapple
- ➤ 1 red onion
- ➤ 2 tomatoes
- ➤ 1 chilli
- ➤ 1 lime
- ➤ 50g lamb's lettuce
- ➤ 150ml boiling water
- ➤ Sea salt
- ➤ 2 tsp olive or coconut oil

Directions

- ➤ Tip the rice into a sieve and give it a good rinse under cold water. Tip it into a small pan. Pour in 150ml boiling water and add a pinch of salt. Pop on a lid, bring to the boil and then turn down the heat under the pan to very low. Gently simmer for 25 mins till the rice has absorbed all the water. Take the pan off the heat and leave it in the pan, lid on, to steam for 5 mins to finish cooking the rice.

➢ Pop the steaks in a dish or on a plate. Mix 2 tsp jerk seasoning with 2 tsp oil to make a paste and then rub it all over the steaks. Set them aside to marinate while you make the pineapple salsa.

➢ Slice the top off the pineapple, then slice it in half. Slice the base and skin off the pineapple half and use the tip of a small, sharp knife to cut out the tough 'eyes'. Finely chop the pineapple flesh and pop it in a bowl.

➢ Peel and finely chop the onion and add it to the pineapple. Dice the tomatoes and add them to the bowl. Halve the chilli, flick out the seeds and white pith (or leave a little in for extra heat) and finely chop the chilli. Add to the bowl.

➢ Finely grate in the zest from the lime
and squeeze in the juice. Add a pinch
of salt and stir to mix. Set to one side.

➢ Put a frying or griddle pan on a high
heat for 3-4 mins till it's smoking hot.
Add the steaks and fry for 30 secs-1
min on each side, depending on how
well done you like your steaks. Slide
them onto a warm plate, loosely cover
with foil and rest for 2 mins.

➢ Fluff the rice with a fork and divide
between 2 warm plates. Arrange
handfuls of the lamb's lettuce on the
plate alongside the rice. Pop a steak on
each plate, spoon over the pineapple
salsa and serve

Loaded Overstuffed Baked Potatoes

TOTAL TIME: 55 MINUTES

INGREDIENTS

- ➤ 4 small to medium size red potatoes washed and pricked with a fork
- ➤ 3 tablespoons butter
- ➤ 1/2 teaspoon salt plus a bit more for sprinkling
- ➤ 1/4 cup sour cream
- ➤ 3/4 cup shredded cheddar cheese
- ➤ 4 tablespoons chopped green onions or chives

DIRECTIONS

- ➤ Preheat the oven to 425
- ➤ While that's heating, cook your potatoes in the microwave until they are tender. For me, that was about 8 to 9 minutes. Cook yours in 3 minute

increments if you aren't sure how long your microwave will take.

➢ When the potatoes are fork tender, remove them to a cutting board and cut off the top about 1/4 the thickness of your potato.

➢ Scoop out the insides, leaving a little bit of potato around the inside.

➢ Transfer to a cookie sheet and divide one tablespoon of butter into fourths.

➢ Add one fourth to the bottom of each potato skin and sprinkle with a tiny bit of salt inside each one.

➢ Bake 15 minutes until the skins are brown and crisp.

➢ While the skins bake, add the remaining 2 tablespoons butter, the sour cream, 1/2 teaspoon salt, and the cheese to the potatoes in the bowl. Mix well with a hand mixer or mash by hand for a chunkier potato.

➢ When the shells are crisp, remove from the oven and transfer the filling into the shells piling it high.

➢ Bake 15 more minutes until golden brown and hot.

➢ Top with green onions and serve warm or room temperature. Freezes well too.

Garlic Herb Cauliflower Rice

TOTAL TIME: 20 MINUTES

Ingredients

➢ 1 medium head cauliflower or 16 ounces store-bought cauliflower rice

➢ 1/2 cup sliced almonds

➢ 2 tablespoons butter or substitute extra virgin olive oil

- 2 cloves garlic, minced
- 1/4 teaspoon fine sea salt
- Freshly ground black pepper, to taste
- 3/4 cup chopped fresh herbs like parsley, dill, cilantro, and basil
- 1 tablespoon lemon juice or more to taste

Directions

- To turn a head of cauliflower into rice, there are two options. Use a food processor or use a box grater.
- If using a food processor, cut the head of cauliflower into medium chunks and remove the core. Working in batches, add the cauliflower to the bowl of a food processor and pulse until the cauliflower is broken down into very small bits that resemble rice.

➢ If using a box grater, cut the head of cauliflower into quarters and remove the core. Use the medium-sized holes to grate each quarter into small bits resembling rice.

➢ Optional step, for the best cauliflower rice, before cooking, transfer the riced cauliflower to a clean dish towel and press to remove excess moisture.

➢ Add the almonds to a large skillet over medium heat. Stir the almonds around the pan until they are fragrant and lightly toasted, about 3 minutes. Keep a close eye on the nuts since they do toast quickly. Transfer the toasted almonds to a bowl and save for later.

➢ Return the skillet to the heat and add the butter. When the butter is melted and bubbling, stir in the garlic. Cook the garlic, stirring it around the pan, until fragrant, about 30 seconds.

➢ Add the cauliflower rice, salt, and a few grinds of black pepper. Cook, stirring every once and a while, until the cauliflower rice is crisp-tender and starts to turn light brown in places, 7 to 10 minutes.

➢ Take the skillet off of the heat, and then stir in the fresh herbs, lemon juice, and toasted almonds. Taste then adjust with additional salt, pepper or lemon juice

Macaroni cheese and greens

TOTAL TIME: 60 MINUTES

Ingredients

➢ 225 g (8oz) macaroni

- 200 g (7oz) green beans, trimmed and halved
- 250 g (9oz) cauliflower, cut into small florets
- 3 tbsp. olive oil
- 50 g (2oz) plain flour
- 600 ml semi-skimmed milk
- 125 g (4oz) extra mature cheddar, finely grated
- 2 tsp. wholegrain mustard
- 100 g (3 ½oz) frozen peas
- 50 g (2oz) kale, shredded

Directions

- Preheat the oven to 180°C (160°C fan) mark 4. Bring a large pan of lightly salted water to boil. Tip in pasta and cook for 5min, add green beans and continue cooking for 2min more, then tip in cauliflower, bring back to boil for a final 2min, until just cooked and still crunchy. Drain.

➢ Meanwhile, heat 2½tbsp olive oil in a large saucepan and whisk in the flour. Cook for 2min, until beginning to smell toasty, then take off the heat. Gradually add the milk, whisking until smooth between each addition. Return pan to the heat and cook for 10min, stirring constantly, until thickened and smooth. Stir in 100g (3½oz) cheese and the mustard. Season.

➢ Add pasta, cooked vegetables and peas to the sauce, stir well. Spoon into 4 mini ovenproof baking dishes. Toss the kale with remaining oil and cheese and scatter over the pasta. Cook in the oven for 15-20min, until bubbling and golden.

CONCLUSION

As you incorporate these nutrient-rich recipes into your daily routine, remember that every positive choice you make contributes to your overall well-being.

Whether it's choosing whole foods, engaging in regular physical activity, or finding effective stress management techniques, each step counts.

Maintaining a healthy lifestyle is a holistic approach that extends beyond the kitchen. It involves cultivating habits that support your body, mind, and spirit. Celebrate the progress you make, no matter how small, and recognize that every effort toward a healthier lifestyle is a step in the right direction.

As you conclude this book, take a moment to reflect on the positive changes you can make and the impact they can have on your health. Embrace the power of nutrition, lifestyle choices, and the support available to you as you move forward on your path to a healthier, happier life.

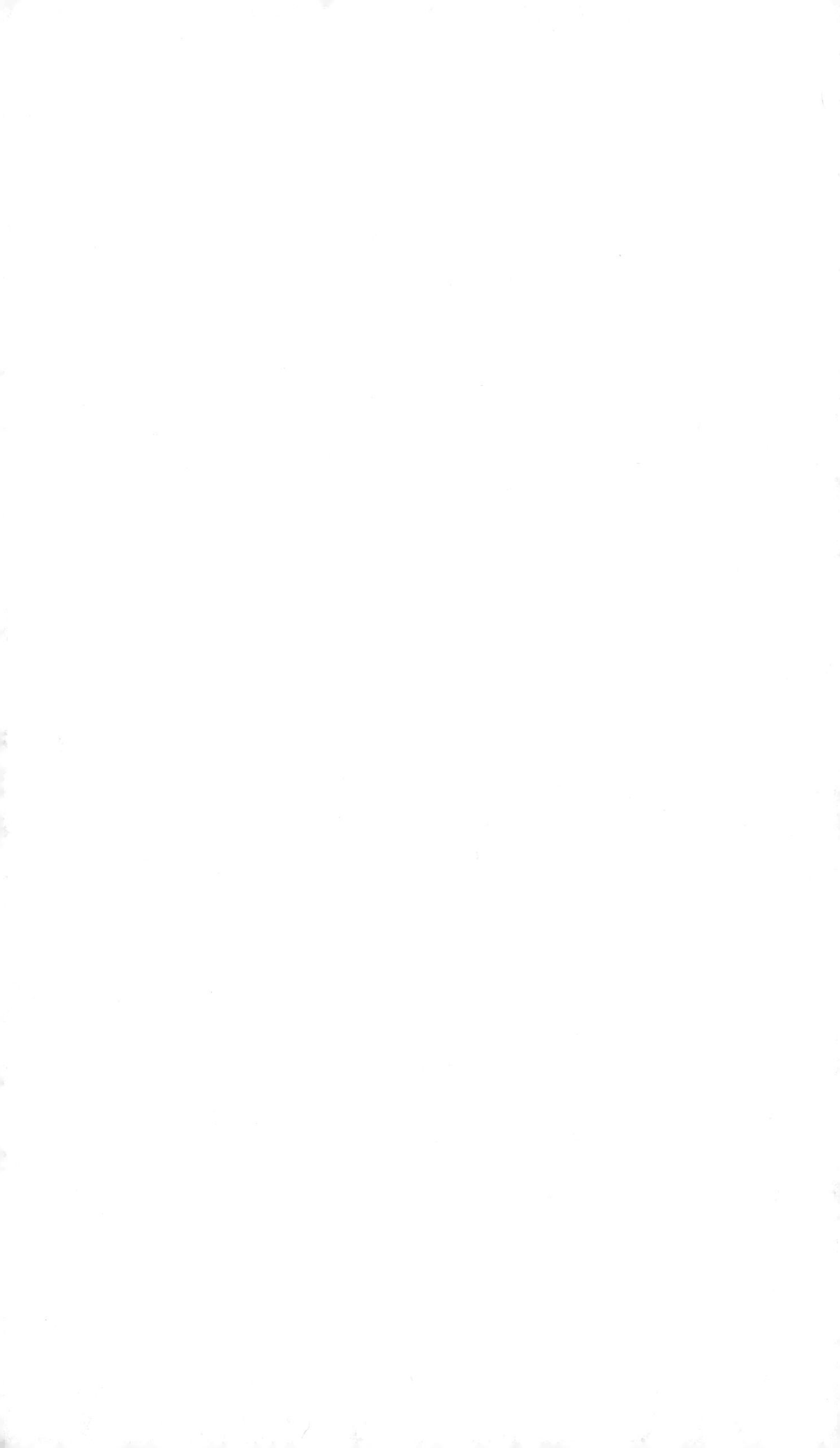

www.ingramcontent.com/pod-product-compliance
Lightning Source LLC
Chambersburg PA
CBHW050746260726
48661CB00001B/441